Alkaline Body: How to Change an Acid Body into an Alkaline Body

"Discover the secret to having a disease free body. This can only be accomplished through having an alkaline body."

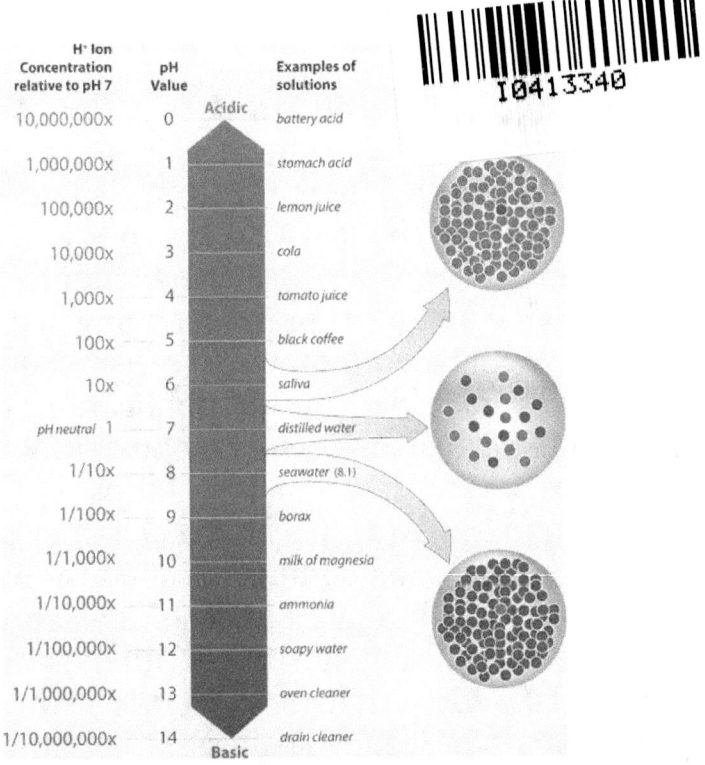

H⁺ Ion Concentration relative to pH 7	pH Value		Examples of solutions
10,000,000x	0	Acidic	battery acid
1,000,000x	1		stomach acid
100,000x	2		lemon juice
10,000x	3		cola
1,000x	4		tomato juice
100x	5		black coffee
10x	6		saliva
pH neutral 1	7		distilled water
1/10x	8		seawater (8.1)
1/100x	9		borax
1/1,000x	10		milk of magnesia
1/10,000x	11		ammonia
1/100,000x	12		soapy water
1/1,000,000x	13		oven cleaner
1/10,000,000x	14	Basic	drain cleaner

By Rudy S. Silva, Natural Nutritionist

Alkaline Body: How to Change an Acid Body into an Alkaline body © 2014 by Rudy S. Silva

ISBN-13: 978-1495240584

ISBN-10: 1495240584

Disclaimer and Terms of Use: The Author and Publisher has strived to be as accurate and complete as possible in the creation of this book, notwithstanding the fact that he does not warrant or represent at any time that the contents within are accurate due to the rapidly changing nature of the Internet. While all attempts have been made to verify information provided in this publication, the Author and Publisher assumes no responsibility for errors, omissions, or contrary interpretation of the subject matter herein. Any perceived slights of specific persons, peoples, or organizations are unintentional. This book is not intended for use as a source of legal, business, accounting health, or financial advice. All readers are advised to seek services of competent professionals in legal, business, accounting, medical and finance field.

Printed in the United States of America

Table of Contents

1: Creating An Alkaline Body

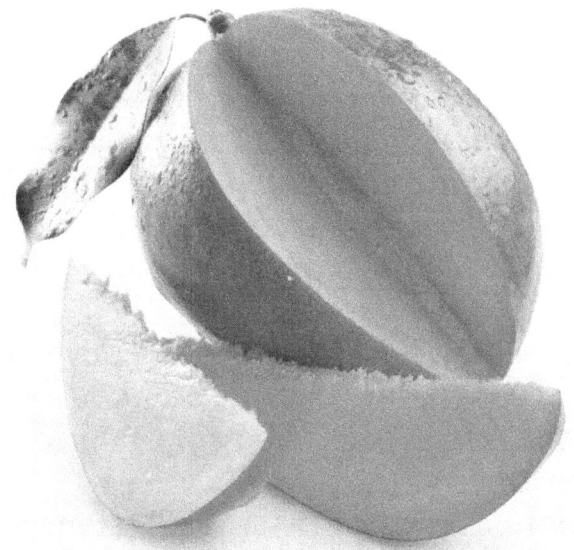

Acids in Your Body

This e-book is all about how you can create an alkaline body. It is well known that most people have an acid body; otherwise, there would not be so much sickness in this world.

If you are sick, have a disease, or don't want to be sick, then, you need the information in this book. To have the best health that you can create comes from bringing your body back to normal, back to where it was intended to be, an alkaline body.

This is not a book about alkaline recipes. You can create this yourself. This book gives you the basics on how you can determine, if you have an acid body, and if you do, how you can change it into an alkaline body.

An acid body is where you have more acid in your body than you can neutralize. When you have an excess of acid floating around in your body, it has a destructive nature. Its detrimental effects are so numerous, it's best to just to say, that your body is headed towards an irreparable condition.

This book is about how to stop your body's acids from destroying cells, tissue, organs, and body systems. It is also about how to stop the pain that goes with this acid destruction.

There is only one way to stop acid, from destroying your body, and this is what you will learn from this book.

Using pH Litmus Paper

You will learn how to monitor your body's acidic condition, using pH litmus paper. You can use this paper to measure your initial body condition and then continue to monitor it, as you apply the changes recommended, in this book.

With litmus pH paper, you can measure your saliva and urine. Using these readings, you can start making changes, in your eating habits. Then you can re-measure your saliva and urine, to see what improvements you have made towards creating an alkaline body.

Nutrition Ideas

What you will learn here is all about nutrition. These ideas will help your understand the foundation of some of the strongest health concepts. These concepts are explained in an easy to understand manner. Here are some of the nutritional and chemical terms that will be used in this book.

Bioelectrical or bioelectrical-chemical
Ions
pH
Acid food
Alkaline foods
Acid waste
Acid body
Alkaline body
Acid Burning Foods and Concepts

To create an alkaline body, you need to burn the acid in your body. This is done by eating certain fruits and vegetables. Once this acid is burned, it is routed out of your body through your elimination channels. You will be given a list of the best fruits and vegetables to eat, which will lead you to creating the best health ever.

Body Cleanse

To get you started in this short program of creating an alkaline body from an acid body, you need to do a short body cleanse. This will get rid of the excess acid, in your body. This is an easy body cleanse that you can finish in 3 to 4 days.

This cleanse will eliminate your constipation, if you have it. It will also cleanse your blood, lymph, and body. It will give you a fresh start, with a minimum of acid in your body. Then with the concepts in this book, you will continue to eliminate the acid waste that is destroying your body.

Body Cycles
There are three body cycles that you have. In the first body cycle, you will discover how to detoxify your body of acids every morning.

In the other cycles, you will learn how to eat your lunch and dinner meals, so that you don't create a lot of body acid.

The Power of Fruits

In the last chapters, you will discover more of why fruits have to the power to cure you, and drugs don't.

These chapters cover the importance of eating and using fruits and vegetables to keep healthy and to recover from sickness. Fruits and vegetables are central, to keep your body alkaline. There are some fruits that are considered acid and some that are alkaline, and you will discover what this really means, and how your body uses these different types of produce.

2: What Is Nutrition About?

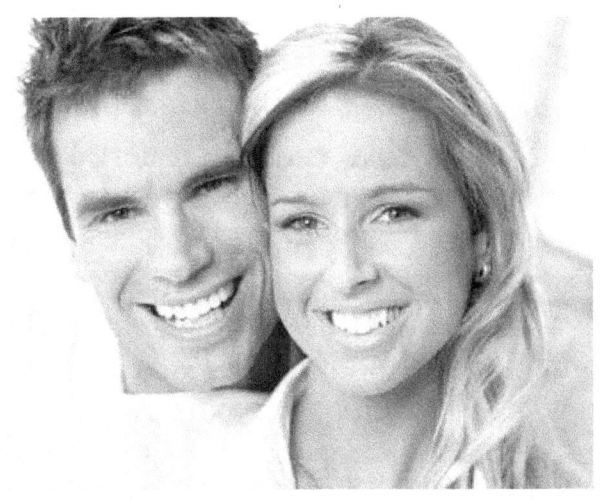

Here is the definition of Nutrition as provided by The Council on Food and Nutrition of the American Medical Association:

"Nutrition is the science of food, the nutrients and the substances therein, their action, interaction, and balance in relation to health and disease, and the process by which the organism ingests, digests, absorbs, transports, utilizes and excretes food substances."

So you can see that nutrition is not a simple matter of eating the right food, but it is also, understanding how food is processed in your body and how it gives you life and health.

By understanding and using nutrition, you can create maximum health.

The amount information that can be covered in this e-book is just a small portion that comes from the science of nutrition. This course concentrates on explaining how, why, and when certain food groups should be eaten for creating the best health possible.

Nutrients – Nutrients are chemicals that come from food and are used to feed your cells. They regulate and control your body processes and provide you with energy. They create new tissue, organ, and bone cells and regulate various chemical activities in your body. Your body is in constant bioelectrical chemical activity, and cells are constantly being created, repaired, or replaced.

There are six groups of nutrients that you eat.

Proteins
Carbohydrates
Water
Fats
Vitamins
Minerals

If you do not provide the nutrients that your body needs to create new replacement cells, your body will use chose other "similar chemicals" to rebuild your cells. Because these "similar chemicals" are not the correct chemicals, the cells that are built will be mutant or un-natural cells. This is why so call "junk food" or processed foods give you poor health - lack nutrients the body can use. Your body needs a tremendous amount of nutrients every day to keep all of your body activities going and for rebuilding your body daily.

Essential Nutrients are chemical substances that your body cannot create or create enough of them. They are nutrients that must come from food. Omega-3 is one such essential nutrient. It cannot be created in the body. If you do not supply it by eating fish, healthy oils, or taking supplements, you will have poor health and will develop painful diseases.

Bioelectrical or bioelectrical-chemical – refers to the chemical reactions that occur in your body. Bio refers to life processes. Bioelectrical is the electrical processes that occur between
ions, electrons, and light (photons), creating voltages and current. Your body is an electric body that forces chemical reactions for creating life and health.

Ions are single elements like silver, gold, calcium, sodium or molecules like a hydroxyl, amino acid, or fatty acid that has an electrical charge associated with it. If it has a negative charge, then it has an excess electron revolving around it so it is unstable and wants to attach itself to another atom or molecule - chemical reaction. If it has a positive charge, then it has an electron or electrons missing, and it also is looking to attach itself to another molecule that can provide those missing electrons.

It is important to know what an ion is, since your body is also bioelectrical and chemical and functions when ions move around in the different fluids of your body and through cell walls. Later, I will be talking about calcium ions, potassium ions, sodium ions, and many other nutrients in ionic form.

Now, let's talking about hydrogen ions or (H) + and Hydroxyl ions or (OH)-. In the next chapters, you will learn about pH and how H+ and OH- are used to determine pH values of liquids. Your whole body revolves around maintaining the pH of the different liquids in your body, so that body control is maintained and health is preserved.

3: Discover The Meaning of pH

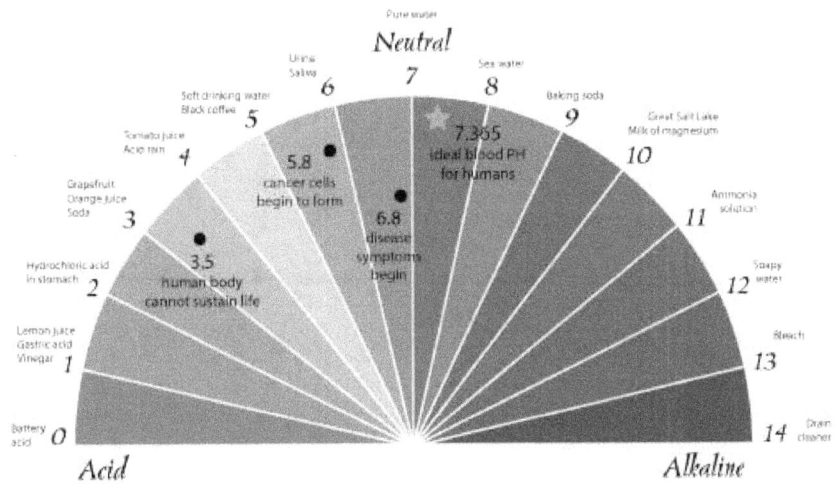

The pH Tests

One of the most important ideas in nutrition is creating an alkaline body so that you can improve your immunity and eliminate illness.

To get started in this quest, you need to determine what kind of body you have, acid or alkaline. Using pH litmus paper you can make this determination.

To find out what your health base line is, you will be doing the following tests below. You need to know what your level of health is, before you start making changes in your life patterns.

You will be doing these tests, as you progress through these outlined steps. This will evaluate how you are doing in your cleansing and new diets. These tests are not exact clinical tests, but they are good enough for checking where you are and how you are progressing.

The three tests you will learn how to use are,

pH saliva test
Lemon pH saliva test
urine test
What is pH testing?

Now, let's talk about hydrogen ions or (H) + and Hydroxyl ions or (OH)-. In the next paragraph, you will learn about pH and how H+ and OH- are used to determine pH values of liquids.

Your whole body revolves around maintaining the pH of different liquids in your body, so that your body remains in good health. When your body pH is not normal, you become sick, your cells start to deteriorate, and you form diseases.

pH – is a complex mathematical and chemical system that was developed to determine when a liquid or solution was an acid or base. The chemical definition of pH is:

"The negative logarithm of the hydrogen ion

molarity"

Since the pH scale is logarithmic, each whole pH value, below 7.0 are ten times more acidic. So, pH 6.0 is ten times more acidic than pH 7.0. pH 5.0 is 100 times more acidic than 7.0, and pH 4.0 is 1000 times more acid than 7.0.

The same holds for base, alkaline, pH values above pH 7.0. But, unlike acids where the pH goes down and the acid strength goes up, the alkaline values above 7.0, increase in strength as their value goes up.

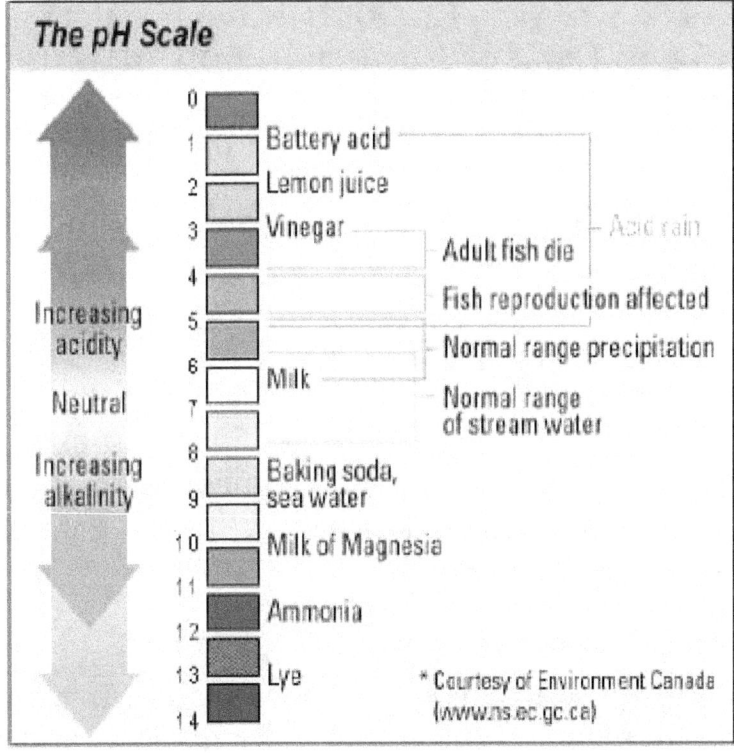

In an alkaline solution, a pH above than 7.0, means

the strength of the alkaline solution is stronger. An alkaline solution of 8.0 is ten times stronger than a solution of 7.0. See the chart below for more information on how pH strength changes from one value to another.

pH Value For Different Substances
A pH of 1 (Stomach Acid) 1,00,000 (H)+ atoms - Acid
A pH of 2 (Lemon Juice) 100,000 (H)+ atoms - Acid
A pH of 4 (Tomato Juice) 1,000 (H)+ atoms - Acid
A pH of 6 (Saliva)............. 10 (H)+ atoms - Acid
A pH of 7 (Water) ....1 (H)+ atoms Neutral
A pH of 8 (Sea Water) .....10 (H)+ atoms - Alkaline
A pH of 10 (Milk of Magnesia) 1,000 (H)+ atoms - Alkaline
A pH of 12 (Soapy Water) 100,000 (H)+ atoms - Alkaline
A pH of 14 (Drain Cleaner) 10,000,000(H)+ atoms – Alkaline

The basic unit of pH is the hydrogen ion, H+. pH is a measure of the amount of Hydrogen ions that exists in a solution. The more hydrogen ions that exist in a solution the more acidic it becomes. In your body, when your lymph liquid is acidic, it is damaging to your cells and tissues.

In your stomach, the pH is highly acidic, 1.5 to 3.0 pH. This pH is necessary to break down protein. But, your stomach lining is highly alkaline and this protects it, from your high stomach acid.

The pH of Water

Water is considered neutral. It is neither an acid nor alkaline and has a pH value of 7.0. This means that water has as many H+ ions as OH- ions. Water's chemical formula is H2O, which is equal to two H+ and one OH-. When chemicals are mixed with water, the mixture can become either acidic or basic.

Liquids, which are Acid or Alkaline

You don't need to understand the mathematics behind pH values, but there it is. What is important is that you understand that a liquid with a pH of 1.0 is very acidic. If you were to put a few drops of this liquid on your hand, it would burn and damage your skin immediately. A pH of 12 is a highly alkaline solution and is not as damaging as acid, but it would still burn your skin.

A pH less than 7 are acidic and a pH greater than 7 is basic. When a liquid is an acid, we call it an acidic solution or an acid solution. When a liquid is alkaline, we called it a basic solution or an alkaline solution. I will be using these terms interchangeably.

Three pH Body Tests

There are three simple tests that you can do with your pH litmus paper. These tests can give you an idea of how acidic or alkaline your body is and how strong your alkaline reserves are. Your alkaline reserves, or body mineral stores, are the amount of minerals you have stored in your body lymph liquid, in tissues, joints, organs, and blood. Most people are low in alkaline reserves and this is why they have a hard time, recovering from a disease.

You will be doing a saliva test, a lemon saliva test, and urine test.

You want your body's internal liquid to be just slightly acidic or just slightly alkaline. In a later chapter, you will find out why your body should be slightly alkaline.

Always record your pH readings to have a historical record. Use an excel spreadsheet or a daily note book.

Many doctors deny the accuracy or use of this pH saliva test and say it is of no value. Frankly, they prefer you to pay them a visit, so that they can put you under their care, but, in an article written by Dr. Steven Zodkoy, A Free and Simple Test for pH, a Potential Health Tester, he promotes the use of this test.

Another important issue related to pH is the oxygen level. Tissue and cells have more oxygen available to them, when your body pH is 7.4 as compared to when it is 6.4. This is very important for acne, because more oxygen throughout your body means fewer parasites and toxic wastes.

It has been found that the average American's tissue pH is between 5.5 and 6.0. This indicates that they have a severe lack of oxygen in their cells and lymph liquid. Lack of oxygen in your body is known to create serious terminal diseases. It is oxygen that destroys all types of bacteria and pathogens that live inside your body and make you ill.

Those of you with acid bodies and that lack cell and lymph oxygen can correct your condition. You can learn what it takes to bring your body back to an alkaline condition. This will give your body a chance to repair tissue and organs, if they have not been severely damaged. How to make your body more alkaline through diet is discussed in a later chapter.

Litmus pH Paper

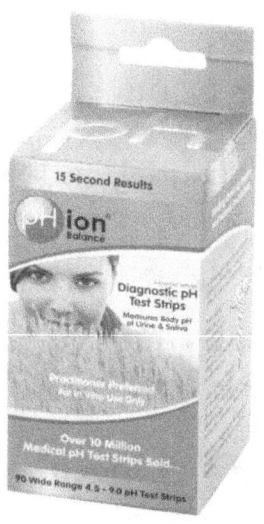

By testing your pH regularly, you can decide the validity of using pH litmus paper, to determine the level of your health. As you go through this program, you can test your saliva and urine to see, if your body has become more alkaline.

You need to take these pH tests for three days for at least two to three times a day to get an average value. This will establish a pH base line or a starting health point for you.

Where to buy pH Litmus Paper

You want to buy the pH paper that gives you accurate readings. Buy the paper that comes in pH increments of 0.2 or 0.25.

You can purchase some pH litmus paper at a drug store, laboratory outlet or through the Internet. Go to Amazon and get this product, <u>PHion Balance Diagnostic pH Test</u> Strips, .25 increments. This is the easiest way to get this pH paper.

Water is considered neutral. It is neither an acid nor alkaline and has a pH of 7.0. What this means is that water has as many H+ ions as OH-, hydroxyl ions. Water's chemical formula is H20, which is equal to two H+ and one OH-. When chemicals are mixed with water, the mixture can become either acidic or basic.

You don't need to understand the mathematics of this definition, but there it is. What is important is that you understand that a pH of 1.0 is very acidic, and if you were to put a few drops on your hand, it would burn and damage your skin immediately.

A pH of 12 is a highly alkaline solution and is not as damaging as acid, but it would burn your skin.

A pH less than 7 are acidic and a pH greater than 7 is basic.

When a liquid is an acid, we call it an acidic solution or an **acid solution**. When a liquid is a base, we called it a basic solution or an **alkaline solution**. I will be using these terms interchangeably.

Acid Forming Food – is food that when metabolized or digested by your cells leave a residue or ash that is acidic. It is this acid that is released by the cell into the lymph liquid where is can move into your tissues or be eliminated through the lymph node, moved into the blood, then to the kidneys and out through the urine. Acid waste can also find its way into the colon for disposal. If this acid waste remains in your tissue or lymph liquid, it will make the pH of that area or liquid acidic.

Unfortunately, acid wastes, in the colon, that are not eliminated are reabsorbed through the colon wall and into the liver and put back into general circulation. This happens when you have constipation and fecal matter travels slowly in the colon. They then deposit in the tissue. It is these residues that determine sickness or health. In a later chapter, you will discover how to eliminate or reduce these harmful acids.

Alkaline Forming food – is alkaline residue or ash that is formed in your cells after it is metabolized or digested. Each food that you eat results in a residue or ash, which changes the surrounding liquid pH in your cells and outside of the cells to an acid liquid or an alkaline liquid. For good health and a clean body, you want to eat those foods that have alkaline wastes, since these alkaline ions can neutralize acid wastes and prevent them from accumulating and causing damage to your body.

The determination of alkaline forming or acidic forming food is not what the pH of the food is before you eat it. An acid food before eating can be an alkaline forming food after it is metabolized by your cells. This concept can be a bit confusing, since you do not normally think about what your food becomes after it's used up by your cells. The left over, after your cell uses the food, you eat always produces a residue that can be acidic or alkaline.

In the following chapters, alkaline forming food is also referred to as acid binding food. It is called this since the alkaline residue or ash will bind with acids so your body can eliminate them.

Acid Body – you are considered to have an acid body if your overall body pH is below 7.0. As your body changes to lower pH values, the more susceptible, you become for creating disease. Here's your sickness level vs. your pH
level. This pH is an average for your saliva and urine readings, which will be covered later.

pH level of around 7.5 – healthy
pH level of 6.0 to 6.5 – not feeling good and are starting to create a disease
pH level of 5.0 to 6.0 - has major health problems
pH level of 4.5 – 5.0 – have a terminal disease

4: Your First Alkaline Tests

The pH Range Chart

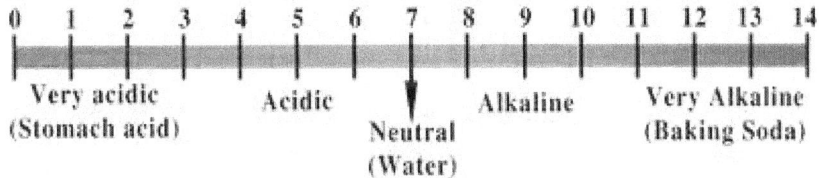

Here are 3 simple tests that you can do with your pH paper. These tests can give you an idea of how alkaline your body is and how strong your alkaline reserves are. Write down your readings and keep track of each test.
Saliva Test

Here is a simple test you can perform on your saliva that will give you an idea of where you stand with your body pH level. Your saliva contains mineral salts that keep it alkaline at 7.4. If your body is deficient in alkaline food or minerals, it will take the minerals from your saliva causing it to drop in pH.

If your saliva is below normal, you can

influence your saliva's pH to read higher, by eating more acid binding (acid binding food will be explained in the next chapter) food and to supplement with potassium, magnesium and calcium.

Keep in mind there are some inaccuracies with this method since your body fluids are always in transition. This test simply gives you an idea of what your saliva pH is at that moment. Use this information for your own education. Then as you begin to change your eating habits and lifestyle, you can retest to see if there is a difference.

Many doctors deny the accuracy or use of this saliva test and say it is of no value. Frankly, they prefer you to pay them a visit so that they can put you under their care, but, in an article written by Dr. Steven Zodkoy, A Free and Simple Test for pH, a Potential Health Tester, he promotes the use of this test.

http://ezinearticles.com/?A-Free-and-Simple-Test-for-pH,-a-Potential-Health-Tester&id=2928

Here's where you can see his resume.

http://www.monmouthadvancedmedicine.co
m/Staff/ZodkoyResume.html

By testing your pH regularly, you can decide
the validity of using pH litmus paper to
determine the level of your health. As you
make changes, you can test your saliva and
urine to see if the pH litmus color changes.

You need to take this test for 3 days and at
least 3 times a day and get an average value so
that you can establish a base line or a starting
point for yourself.

Purchase some pH litmus paper at a drug
store, laboratory outlet or order it through the
Internet. The better pH paper you can buy is
on Amazon, with a .25 increment in pH
change.

Starting Your Saliva Testing

Gather saliva in your mouth then swallow. Do
this two times.

Place the pH paper under your tongue. Let it
sit there for 5 seconds to wet it and then

remove it. Let it sit for 20 seconds, compare the color of your pH paper to the color chart on the bottle and record the pH.

Do this test around one hour before eating or around two hours after eating. This reading gives you an idea about the state of your saliva. Your first test should be done first thing in the morning, before you rinse out your mouth or drink anything.

Saliva and Lemon Test

Now, do this test immediately after you do your saliva test above. Squeeze half of lemon juice in one ounce of water and swish it around in your mouth for 5 seconds or so then spit it out, wait one minute now, measure your mouth's pH with litmus paper. Just place the paper into your mouth and wet it.

Now compare the color and pH value of this reading with your first pH saliva reading. This reading should have a higher alkaline reading than your first saliva reading.

Good Saliva Test

If this reading has a higher alkaline reading, it means you have alkaline reserves. The higher the alkaline reading you have the stronger your alkaline reserves. A small alkaline upward change means you have alkaline reserves, but they are not as strong as they should be.
For example,

- Morning reading is 6.5 pH (the higher the better)
- After the lemon test reading 6.9 pH

These readings are good, and indicate you have some body mineral stores. But your Morning reading of 6.5 is a little low and should be closer to 7.0 for better health.

Weak Saliva Test

If your pH reading does not change from your first reading or actually goes down by becoming more acidic, then your alkaline reserves are weak, and you need to make some major changes in the way you eat. In this course, you will see what you will need to do to bring up your alkaline reserves, so that you will not be susceptible to serious diseases.

Now, suppose your readings were,

- First reading 6.5
- Lemon test reading 6.2

There is a drop in your lemon pH, and this is not too good. This means that you don't have enough minerals in your body to neutralize the acid in your mouth. You will have to eat more acid binding food.

Saliva Test Summary

Again, if your lemon test readings have a higher pH reading than your first reading, it means you have alkaline reserves. The bigger the difference between your first test and second test, the stronger your alkaline reserves. A small alkaline upward change means you have alkaline reserves, but they are not as strong as they should be.

If your lemon pH reading does not change from your first reading or actually goes down by becoming more acidic, then your alkaline reserves are weak, and you need to make some major changes in the way you eat. This also means you have a highly acidic body that can create some serious illness, especially if your lemon test pH is down to 6.0 and below.

Urine pH test

There have been clinical studies indicating that urine pH is an accurate reflection of your body responding to the production acid waste.
Each time you test your urine, note what you eat in your evening meal. Eating a high-protein meal, which is an acid meal, will require more alkaline ash to neutralize your acid dinner. If you eat a meal high in vegetables and little protein, then your body should easily neutralize your meal by morning.

Here's how to do the urine pH test

In the morning when you urinate, allow it to flow for a second and then wet your pH litmus paper with urine.

If your urine pH is below 6.0 or 5.8, this indicates that your body did not have enough alkaline ash or ions to neutralize your evening dinner. In addition, you do not have enough alkaline mineral reserves to protect your body from acid damage to your cells and tissues.

If your urine is down to 5.8, this is on the low side, but is considered ok. But, this is not a good place for your pH to be at all the times. You want your urine pH to be close to 6.5. This shows that you have plenty of mineral stores to neutralize a previous night's acid dinner – meat or carbohydrates.

Normal Urine Range is 5.8 to 6.5

A good urine range is from 6.0 and 6.5, indicating that your alkaline reserves are in good shape. Of course, the closer you are to 6.5, the better and this is the pH you should strive for.

High Urine pH

If your morning urine is over 7.2 and higher, this indicates your body is going into an emergency state, using ammonia from the liver in an effort to reduce your acid body. You may read as high as 8.0 indicating for sure you are producing ammonia to neutralize your acid dinner. To change this will require a substantial change in your eating habits. Sometimes you can smell that your urine is ammonia like.

Keep in mind that this may be temporary, but if you consistently see high urine pH, then you definitely have a problem and need to back off from eating acid food.

Test Your Urine for 3 days

Test your urine for 3 days to see if it remains consistent. Record this information to see how it changes as you progress through this program.

- Measure your saliva pH in the morning.
- Measure your morning urine
- Measure your urine pH two times during the day.
- Measure your urine mid-day, two hours after eating

If you're initial pH tests indicate that you have an acid body, then depending on how acidic it is this will determine how long you have work to change your body's acid levels.

Compute the pH Average

After three or four days of saliva and urine readings, you want to take the average of all readings. Here is how you can determine what your pH readings mean.

pH level of 6.5 to 7.4 - You are at a healthy level. However, the higher number is better.

pH level of 6.0 to 6.5 – You may not be feeling good and need to make some changes in your diet.
pH level of 5.0 to 6.0 - You have major health problems.

pH level of 4.5 – 5.0 – You have a terminal disease.

You are considered to have an alkaline body, if your overall body pH liquids are 6.5 to 7.4. This is the pH level that you should strive for. Higher pH values of 7.5 to 8.5 and up are considered detrimental.

Children with an acid body will respond quickly to good changes in eating habits, whereas adults, depending on age, can see results in 5 weeks and up to a year.

A pH Guide

Here is a guide line to what your saliva and urine pH should be.

- Saliva should be 6.6 to 7.4
- Urine should be 5.8 to 6.4

If your urine is down to 5.8, this is ok, since it shows that you are getting rid of body acids. But, you don't always want to have such a low reading. For saliva, a good reading is 6.8.
pH and Oxygen

Another important issue related to pH is the oxygen level. Tissue and cells have more oxygen available to them when your body pH is 7.4 as compared to when it is 6.4.

It has been found that the average American's tissue pH is between 5.5 and 6.0. This indicates that they have a severe lack of oxygen in their cells and lymph liquid. Lack of oxygen in the body is known to create serious terminal diseases. It is oxygen that destroys all types of bacteria and pathogens that live inside your body and make you ill.

Those of you with acid bodies and that lack cell and lymph oxygen can correct your condition by learning what it takes to bring your body back to an alkaline level. This will give your body a chance to repair tissue and organs, provided, they have not been severely damaged.

5: How Minerals Burn Acid

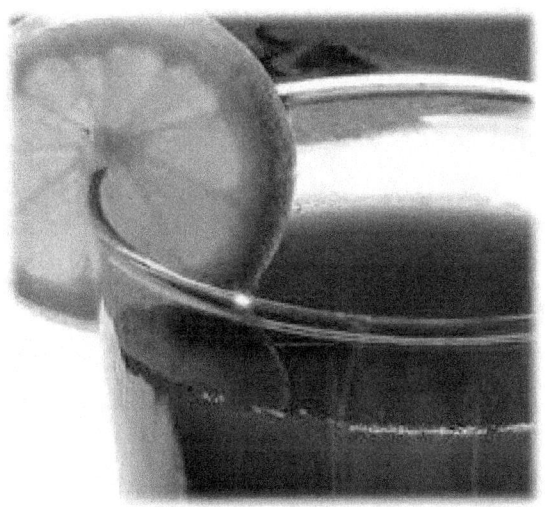

Minerals

Moving your body more toward alkalinity is what will give you the best curative effects of fruits. An alkaline body prevents your body from becoming ill and forming deadly diseases, like all kinds of joint problems, organ degradation, body pain, or even cancer. If you are already sick, then all the chemicals inside fruits will help to revive you to better health. This is provided that your tissue damage has not gone beyond repair.

The minerals most important in changing and

maintaining your body in an alkaline condition are sodium, potassium, chloride, calcium, phosphorus, magnesium, and sulfur.

Now, how your body can become alkaline might become a little confusing at first because of the terms used, but let's break this down into small parts. This process has been discussed in previous chapters, but this explanation gives more details. First, we are going to be defining some terms, so we can then start talking the same language.

Acid Binding

There are certain minerals that are called acid binding. And these are minerals, as mentioned earlier, are the most important ones in fruits, Sodium, potassium, chloride, calcium, phosphorus, magnesium, because they are acid binding.

What acid binding means is when you eat fruits with these minerals, your cells, after metabolism, create an alkaline ash. This ash will seek out acids in your body and bind with them to neutralize them.

Alkaline Ash

Now, that this alkaline forming ash has tied up an acid it is carried to the kidney where it is expelled as urine.

Different reactions can occur when an acid binding

mineral, like say sodium, encounters an acid. Of course, acids in the body are toxic, so the body has the priority of getting rid of them fast, since they can damage tissue and cause pain and disease.

Here is another path way of the acid binding mineral process when it combines with an acid.

The Acid Binding Mineral Process

When you eat acid binding food, the blood carries it to the cells where it is oxidized, digested, or metabolized. The result of this digestion is a carbonic acid salt of alkaline minerals, which reacts with body acids and binds with them. In this process, a weak carbonic acid is created. Now, this weak carbonic acid is taken by the blood into the lungs where it is released as carbon dioxide and water.

If not all the acid toxins are captured by acid binding matter, the remaining acids can be neutralized by body stores of alkaline minerals. If you don't have a good store of alkaline minerals, then these acids will remain in your body creating pain and disease.

But if you do have a good store of alkaline minerals, then these minerals will find these acids, capture them and bind with them. Then these acids are routed out through your urine or colon and out of your body.

So you can see the importance of getting a lot of

alkaline minerals into your body. Without them, acids which do not get bonded to alkaline minerals would move back into body tissue and continue their body damage.

Alkaline Binding

Now, there are also minerals that become alkaline binding and these minerals are sulphur, chlorine, iodine, phosphorous, bromine, fluorine, copper, and silicon.

It is these minerals that when digested by a cell will produce an acid salt that will bind with alkaline minerals. These minerals will be excreted through your urine. When alkaline minerals are bonded to an acid salt, the alkaline mineral is removed from your body, and your body becomes more acidic, the condition you are trying to avoid.

Although you need to eat both foods that are acid binding or alkaline binding, you want to eat more of the acid binding foods.

Keeping Healthy

One of the most important parts of health is keeping the lymph liquid around your cells clean and free of toxins. To do this you need provide alkaline minerals to occupy the lymph liquid, and you need to remove the acids that accumulate in that liquid and in all parts of your body tissue. You can do this by detoxifying your body and providing alkaline minerals for your lymph liquid.

Body Detoxification

The highest priority of the body is to detoxify itself. One of the best ways to help your body detoxify is to provide minerals that bind with acids that are in the cells, tissues, organs, and muscles. What these alkaline acid binding minerals do is to pull out the toxins that are dispersed throughout your body.

With the help of the liver which detoxifies the blood, the kidney that removes impurities from the blood and the lungs which removes the CO_2 which results from alkaline acid binding, your body is constantly detoxifying itself. However, when it is over loaded with acid toxins from your lifestyle, a complete detox of your body becomes impossible.

Where do Acid Toxins Come From?

So why is the body overloaded with toxins? Why can't the liver take care of these toxins? The liver has the function to remove acid wastes from natural food that is created by food digestion and cell metabolism. When it encounters acid wastes such as food enhancers, dyes, preservatives, pesticides, and the variety of additives, the liver does not always know how to break them down to make them harmless.

But your body does not give up so easily when it knows that the liver was not able to disintegrate food additives. What it does is it instructs calcium to bind with these toxic acids and to take them far away from the blood stream. The result is that calcium binding with acid forms a deposit, and this deposit can be placed in your teeth, your joints, and as bone spurs, which grow in your feet or shoulders, vertebra, or muscle tissue. These calcium deposits are very painful, and if you have ever experienced them, you know how much.

Now, we have talked about acid toxins in the body that are brought in through food and the environment. But there is another factor that creates acid in the body and that is emotions that are occur through life stresses, like work pressures, divorce, friendship problems, martial issues, and other similar problems. These emotional problems create acidic molecules that embed themselves into your tissues just like food acids.

Body Organs

All body organs function to rid the body of acid waste or toxins. Lack of alkaline binding food causes deterioration of the function of these organs. Each organ has a specific function in the elimination and neutralization of acid wastes, and it does this in conjunction with alkaline acid binding minerals.

6: Fruits and Vegetable That Neutralize Body Acids

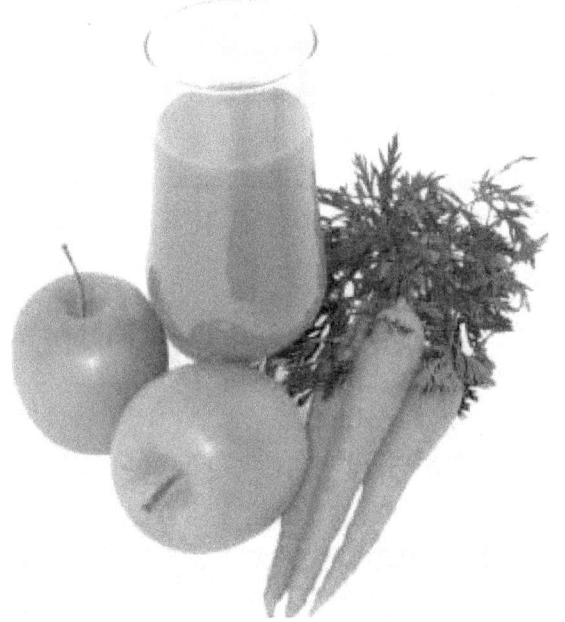

Acid Binding Fruits and Vegetables

Here is a list of fruits, vegetables and other foods that have the highest alkaline minerals and the highest acid production. The percentage number next to these foods indicates the strength of the alkaline minerals or the acid minerals. The closer to 100% the more effective these foods are as an acid reducing food. However you should be eating all foods throughout the list not just the ones at the top of the list.

The percentage assigned to these fruits is based on fresh fruits and vegetables that are organic and not cooked, canned or mixed with sugar. If they are cooked or otherwise processed in some fashion, this will slightly reduce their effectiveness as an acid binding. However, they will still be effective in acid binding.

Acid Binding Fruits with Alkaline Minerals

In the list below are fruits and vegetables with alkaline minerals that create acid binding salts in your body, used to neutralize acid wastes. Foods above 50% in value are more acid binding, which means they will more trap or bind with acid wastes. Foods below 50% are more acid producing and are called alkaline binding, since they tie up or bind with alkaline minerals.

To create an alkaline body, you need to eat 80% acid binding food and 20% alkaline binding food. Work towards this end and you will slowly move your body from acid to alkaline.

Here is the list of foods to eat in the order of priority.

Fruits

Fruits at 100% Acid Binding – Best fruits To Eat

Lemons, melons – any type, watermelon

Fruits at 93% Acid Binding – Great fruits To Eat

Cantaloupes, dried dates, dried figs, limes, mango, papaya

Fruits at 87% Acid Binding – Still Great Fruits To Eat

Kiwis, passion fruit, pineapples, raisins, umeboshi plums

Fruits at 80% Acid Binding – Eat These Fruits

Apricots, avocados, bananas, fresh dates, fresh figs, currants, gooseberries grapes, grapefruits guavas, kumquats, nectarines, pears, persimmons, quince, berries, cactus

Fruits at 73% Acid Binding – Still Fruits To Eat

Apples, oranges, peaches, pomegranate, raspberries, sour grapes, strawberries, carob

Fruits at 67% Acid Binding – Still Neutralizes Acids

Cherries, fresh coconut

Herbal Teas From Leaves at 73% to 86% acid binding

Alfalfa, mint, sage, spearmint, raspberry strawberry comfrey

All Herbs and Spices at 67% to 73% Acid Binding
Fruits At 40% to 47% - Eat less of these fruits

Blueberries, cranberries, plums, prunes

All Fruit Juices From A Juicer 100% Acid Binding

Vegetables

Here is the list of vegetables to eat in order of priority. All of these vegetables will neutralize acid, since they contain minerals that are acid binding.

Vegetables at 93% Acid Binding – best vegetables to eat

Kelp, Seaweed, Watercress, Asparagus

Vegetables at 80% Acid Binding – Still the best to eat

Lettuce Leaf, Oyster plant, Pumpkin, Spinach, Squash, Peas, Carrots, Celery, Chard, Swiss, Dandelion greens

Vegetables at 73% Acid Binding – Great vegetables to eat

Bamboo shoots, Beets, Broccoli, Cabbage, Cauliflower, Collards, Corn, sweet, Ginger (fresh), Mushrooms, Mustard greens, Onions, Pepper, Potatoes, Green, Lima, String, Potatoes

Vegetables at 67% Acid Binding – eat plenty of these

Brussell sprouts, Cucumbers, Eggplant, Okra, Onions, Radishes, Tomatoes

Vegetable juices at 80% to 93% Acid Binding

Parsley, wheat grass, carrot, celery, etc.

Soy Bean Products at 60% Acid Binding – limit your use of tofu since it is a genetically modified organism, GMO

Dried beans, Soy cheese, Soy milk, Tempeh, Tofu

Here are some other misc. foods to eat that are acid binding.

Starches at 80% Acid Binding

Arrowroot flour

Sugar at 73% acid Binding

Honey

Nuts and Seeds at 60 % to 67% Acid Binding

Almonds, sesame seeds, Granola, Essene Bread, Chestnuts

Misc. foods at 60% Acid Binding

Horseradish, Amaranth, Millet, Quinoa, Dried beans, Soy cheese, Soy milk,

The following foods are alkaline binding, which means that they create acids that will bind with alkaline salts and remove them from your body. These foods when eaten in excess will create an acid body. You should only eat around 20% of these foods in your diet, and the other 80% should come from fruits and vegetables or foods that are acid binding. When you eat with this 20/80 formula, you will have an alkaline body.

NOTE: The lower the alkaline binding percentage, the more that food is acid producing.

All oils are basically at 50% and are considered neutral.

This includes almond, avocado, canola, coconut, corn castor, olive, soy, sunflower oil, and etc.

Beans, starches, and nuts and seeds at 40% to 46%
Alkaline Binding

Aduki, Black, Broadbean, Garbanzo, Mung, Pinto, Barley, Corn Meal, Lentils, Brans, Cashews, Coconut (dried), Pecans, Brans, Millet, Filberts, Walnuts, Pumpkin, Sunflower

Starches at 26 to 33 % Alkaline Binding
Brown Rice, Buckwheat, Oats, Spelt, Wheat Whole, Peanuts, corn, rye

Rice at 20% Alkaline Binding
White rice

Sugar at 13% Alkaline Binding
White beet or cane sugar

Meat and Fish

Meat at 26% alkaline binding
Fish With fins and scales, Shellfish - shrimp, scallops, crab lobster, oyster

Meat at 20% Alkaline Binding
Chicken, turkey, rabbit

Meat at 13% Alkaline Binding
Beef, goat, pork, lamb

All oils are basically at 50% and are considered neutral.
This includes almond, avocado, canola, coconut, corn castor, olive, soy, sunflower oil, and etc.

Misc. Products at 13% to 26% Alkaline Binding
Liquor, wine, beer, coffee, black tea, caffeine drinks

7: A Fast Body Cleanse For Acid Burning

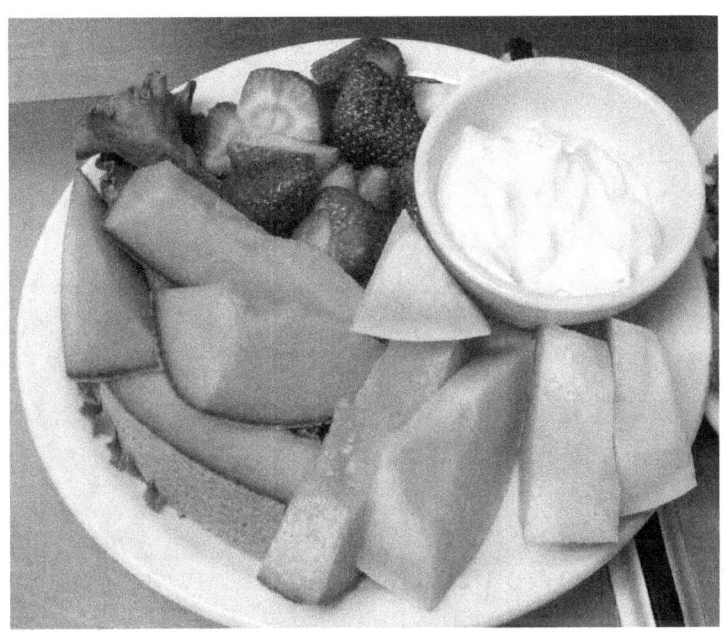

An Easy Body Cleanse

In any health program, the first thing, you need to do is do a colon cleanse. Once you do this, whatever health program you start, you will get the maximum benefits of a new program. To keep good health, you need to make sure you have regular bowel movements. If you are not regular, you will have a toxic colon that will be supplying toxicity to all parts of your body.

This is a relatively easy cleanse to do and will help you eliminate a lot of body waste, which is acidic.

This is a colon, blood, and body cleanse you can do with fruits and vegetable for a 3 to 4 day cleanse.

Constipation

If you eat 3 meals each day, you should have 2 bowel movements a day. If you only have one, then you are short 1 bowel movement.

Normally, if you have 3 full meals a day, you should have 3 bowel movements a day. Don't be fooled by anyone that says one bowel movement in one or two days is ok. This is not true.

If you want to learn how to keep regular using natural remedies, then you can check out my e-book called, "Constipation Natural Cures" Look for it on Google Search or get The Best Constipation Remedies kindle e-book.

So let's get started.

To get your bowels moving like they should, you need to, clean out what is in your colon right now. So the first day is for cleaning out your colon. The next two days is for cleaning the colon and to detoxify the body.

Doing a colon cleanse of a minimum of three days is the best way to start cleaning out the colon, to detoxify the blood, and rejuvenate your body. Just doing a cleanse for three days is not a cure all, and it will require more work on your part by starting to eat more natural foods.

I consider this a mini-fruit juice cleanse. This is to start your body detoxifying. You can do this juice fast once a month for 2-3 days but leave out the prune juice and just drink the juices for 2-3 days. This gives your stomach, small and large intestine and liver a rest and a chance to rejuvenate.

Doing a juice cleanse can give you some side effects where you feel nauseated or slightly sick. Not everyone will get these effects.

This three day colon cleansing is outlined in my "Colon And Blood Cleansing Diet" in kindle form.

In her extensive book, Cooking For Healthy Healing, 1991,

Linda Rector-page, N.D., Ph.D., talks about what a fast does, "Fasting works by self-digestion. During a cleanse, the body in its infinite wisdom, will decompose and burn only the substances and tissue that are damaged, diseased, or unneeded, such as abscesses, tumors, excess fat deposits, and congestive wastes. Even a relatively short fast can accelerate elimination from the liver, kidneys, lungs and skin, often causing dramatic changes as masses of accumulated waste is expelled. Live foods and juices can literally pick up dead matter from the body and carry it away."

Day before the fast

The day before the fast, eat a large salad and two apples. This will give you plenty of fiber to scrub the walls of your colon as you move fecal matter out of your colon the following day.

First day of colon cleanse

Do this cleanse on a Saturday, Sunday or any other day that you don't have to go anywhere.
You will be going to the bathroom all day, and at times you need to be there quick.

Buy the following items.

Organic apple juice – one gallon
Organic apples – 6 for one day
Organic prune juice – one quart
When you first wake up in the morning, drink,
8 oz. of prune juice
10 minutes later drink another 8oz of prune juice
10 minutes later again drink another 8 oz. of prune juice
wait 20 minutes than drink 8 oz. of apple juice
wait 30 minutes than drink another 8 oz. of apple juice

If you haven't sped to the bathroom yet, you will in a little while.

Now you will drink 8 oz. of apple juice every hour until the end of the day. You can stop drinking apple juice around 5 pm.

During the day, you can eat three apples in the morning and 3 apples in the evening.

This process will clean out any fecal matter that has been sitting your colon for days and gets you ready for the next step.

Second Way To Start The Colon Cleanse

Another way to start a colon cleanse is to use a product that is called "Oxy-Powder." This product is in capsules and is used for 30 days. Simply, by taking capsules every day, you will clean out your colon and any build up along your colon walls.

This is a very effective product and will send you to the bathroom frequently as it cleanse out your colon. Start this cleanse on a Saturday so you can have Saturday and Sunday free to start cleaning out your colon.

For a gentle cleanse you can start with about 4 Oxy-Powder capsules. Ten capsules will surely send you to the bathroom frequently. Take the capsules the night before you start your cleanse.

After two days of intense cleaning, you can back off and continue to take a lower capsule dose and continue to cleanse at a slower pace – 4 to 5 capsule per day.

You can get Oxy-Powder on the internet.

Second day of the colon cleanse

During the second day, you can drink different kinds of juice and eat 2-6 apples. You can drink any kind of juice be it fruit or vegetable. A combination of fruit and vegetable juice is good.

Third day of the colon cleanse

The third day is like the second day where you can drink different kinds of juice and eat 2-6 apples or other fruit. You can drink any kind of juice be it fruit or vegetable. A combination of fruit and vegetable juice is good.

Fourth Day, after the fast is done

After you have finished your three-day fast, start eating soft foods to gently adjust your system to food. Here are some of the foods you can eat during the fourth day out of your fast,

Baked potato

Fruit salad

Fruit smoothie

Light soup

Oatmeal, multigrain cereal with banana
Salad
Natural Yogurt

8: Body Cycles That Rid You Of Daily Acids

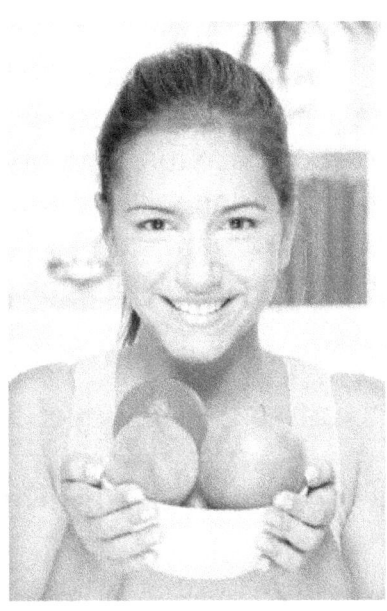

Most of you are looking for ways to improve your health, lose weight, or get rid of an illness that you have. Here's some information that will help you achieve these results. It is called "Using Your Natural Body Cycles" for achieving maximum health. Getting in tune with your Natural Body Cycles requires a change in the way you eat.

Since all of us are addicted to the way we eat, it is, sometimes, difficult to change these habits. But, if you are serious about what you want, this is best information; I have found that will give you good health.

Here is a chance to use the information in the chapter "Fruits And Vegetable That Neutralize Body Acids"

Using your natural body cycle, you will gain better health. But, as you apply body cycles, you might experience side effects, because you will be eliminating more body toxins and body wastes. The side effects may be headaches, stomach upsets, body pain, or similar types of symptoms. These conditions will not last and will disappear as you get rid of more toxins.

Here are the 3 natural body cycles:

Cycle 1 time period: 4 a.m. to noon

This cycle is the time where your body is eliminating toxins, acids, wastes, and derby by urine, bowel movements, and other secretions.

During the elimination cycle, 4 a.m. to noon, eat and drink only fruits and their juices or drink vegetable juices. For breakfast eat a bowl of fruit or have a fruit smoothie made with apple juice and fruits in season. Before noontime eat fruits as a snack. Forty-five minutes before noon eat your last fruit. You can eat and drink all the fruits and juices you want up to noontime.

By eating in this way you are assisting your body's

elimination cycle. This helps your body to eliminate toxins and acids from your body and blood. It is these toxins and acids that make you sick and overweight. Acids are the main cause of most illnesses, and so you want to have an alkaline body. Fruits and vegetables give you an alkaline body.

It takes ½ hour or so to digest fruit and fruit juices. Because of this, they help to cleanse your body of waste. Fruits are 70% water just like your body, and this gives them the cleansing action they have and that your body needs.

Cycle 2 time period: noon to 8 p.m.

This is the time when your body should be taking in food and digesting. During this period, it is time to eat solid foods. What you eat has to be in alignment with what your stomach can do.

Your stomach can only work on one solid food at a time, so your lunch and dinner should only have one solid food. A lunch can consist of chicken and a green salad, fish and a green salad, tuna and a green salad, shrimp and a green salad, beef and a green salad.

Any eating habit that disrupts cycle 2, the eating and digestion cycle, affects the other cycles. Here's how you can help your body's cycle 2 to be more effective.

Eat only one solid food with vegetables during lunch or dinner. Lunch can be one meat or seafood with a fresh vegetable salad.

Limit the amount of water you drink during your eating. Excess water will dilute your digestive acids and slow down digestion of your food.

Eliminate drinking any sodas, coffee, tea or other drinks during your meals. If you need to clear your dry throat use a little water, which is a room temperature. Cold liquids will slow down your digestive processes.

Eating meals with more than one solid food such as meat and potatoes, chicken and rice, fish and rice, chicken and noodles, eggs and toast, cheese and bread will diminish the energy you need during the elimination cycle 1.

It is permissible to eat beef and chicken at the same time but not chicken and eggs or beef and nut or chicken and beans. Eat the same type of protein at the same time but do not mix different proteins.

It's ok to eat different types of carbohydrates at the same time, with a salad, but not with protein, since carbohydrates digest easier than protein.

Eating the right combinations of foods at mealtime helps to preserve your energy for the elimination cycle and prevents you from creating spoiled food in your stomach that is converted to acid waste. It is this acid waste that results in down with various illnesses that terminate their lives early or gain excessive weight.

Cycle 3 time period: 8 p.m. to 4 a.m.

This is the time your body is absorbing and using the food you have eaten during the 12 noon to 8 p.m. period. This is the time the food you have eaten during the day is assimilated, absorbed and distributed throughout your body through your blood.

Food that was eaten during cycle II and that was combined and eaten properly will digest within 3 hours. Whereas food not combines properly, a meal consisting of protein and carbohydrates will take up to 8 hours to pass through the stomach. During this time, your food will putrefy and ferment and become acidic. Under these conditions, you will not get any nutrients from that meat.

Eat your last meal by 6-7 pm so that your food digests in your stomach by the time you go to bed. After three hours later, your food will have moved into your small intestine where it is ready for assimilation.

When you go to bed 3 hours after your last meal, the next 6 hours, until 4am, your body will be absorbing the food you have eaten the previous day.

Remember, anything you do different than what these cycles call for will disrupt them and cause them to become extended. When this happens, your food turns into acid, you don't absorb the value of your food, you lose energy and become tired, and over time, you gain weight and create serious illnesses.

9: Secret Diet Fruit Tips

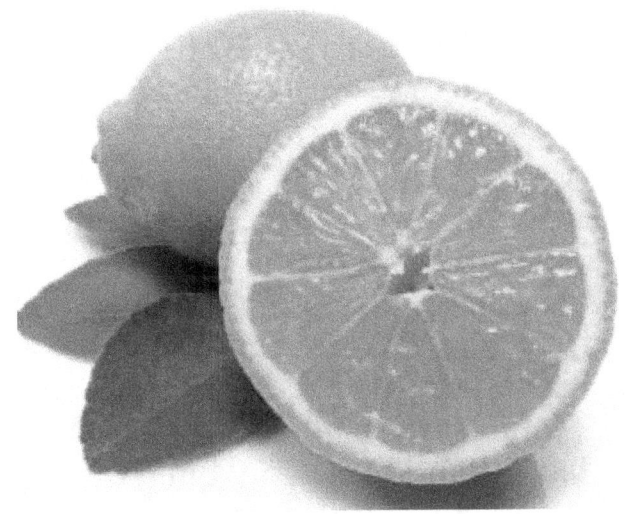

Did you know that there are certain fruits you should be eating to make your body more alkaline? These fruits have the chemicals and elements that transform tissues, cells, and organs into an alkaline condition. This is one of the basic functions of fruits.

Fruits and their juices also have curative powers for preventing and eliminating illness and disease.

Lemon Power

For example, you would think that eating fresh lemons would be creating an acid condition in your body. But it's really the opposite. Lemons contain citric acid, but when your body uses this acid, the result is an alkaline ash residue that binds with acid to move your overall body to a more alkaline level.

In this e-book, you will find ways to use lemons with other fruits to maximize the alkaline effect of these foods. By using lemons at certain times of the day, you will give yourself a boost in your health.

Fruits have the power to bring your body back into the normal range of health. This is because many of the activities you do during the day, you create body acids and fruits can balance out these acids. If you do not neutralize these acids, they will build up in your body and attract and create disease. The number of diseases that result from acid build in your body encompasses practically all diseases.

Body Acids Reabsorbed

If body acids, which are created during digestion or during fecal matter elimination, are not neutralized or eliminated, they can be reabsorbed into your body from the small intestine and colon.

These acids go from the colon into the blood stream and then into the liver. Then, from there they get back into your lymph liquid and deposit themselves into your body tissues.

Mineral Binding

The only way to reduce the detrimental effects of

these acids on your body is to mix them with an alkaline liquid. This is where fruits and vegetables come in. They have the power to provide what is known as "mineral binding," which helps to neutralize the effect of excess body acids or excess alkaline compounds. But in this e-book, we are mainly concerned with the toxic acids that you have in your body.

In addition to reducing or eliminating an acidic body condition, fruits contain 100s of chemicals known and unknown. The chemicals are minerals, vitamins, phytonutrients, anti-oxidants, bioflavonoids, and other natural nutrients.

It's these different chemicals that help you to cure certain body ills. The thing to remember when using fruits to cure is you have to use more of them compared to when you are just eating them for breakfast, lunch or snacks.

With each fruit discussed, you are given ways that you can use them to improve your health.

10: The Fantastic Acid Burning Nutrients In Fruits

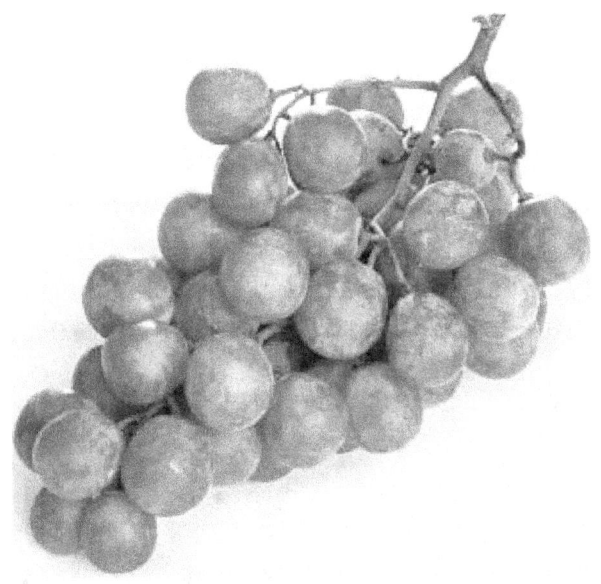

Because fruits are naturally grown from the soil, they pull minerals from the ground and can be a great source of nutrients for you, if the soil is heavy with minerals. Because of these minerals and other nutrients, Fruits have amazing curative effects, when they are eaten raw. In some cases, it is better to cook them for their healing effects.

The best fruits to eat are those that allow your body to become more alkaline. Your body naturally seeks to be in an alkaline condition. In this condition, your body has less pain, inflammation, and disease. It has more energy, and your body is not deteriorating as fast as when your body is filled with acid.

It's ok to eat fruits that make your body acid. However, eating more fruits that make your body alkaline is necessary. This is because most people have an acid body and need to move it to an alkaline condition. Later when you become more alkaline, you will be eating 80% alkaline fruits and 20% acid fruits.

Your body uses minerals to neutralize acids and, in other chemical body reactions, to create simple or complex chemicals that your body needs. So, the body holds specific minerals in a certain way. It holds minerals in "storage" and releases them when they are needed for certain chemical reactions. The storage locations of minerals are in the blood, in organs, in cells, in tissue, and in the liquid inside and outside your cells.

Fruit Benefits

Fruits contain a variety of nutrients that are necessary for maintaining life. Each nutrient has is function in the body. Many of the functions are known, and many are not. Here is a list of some of the main known nutrients and what they do in your body.

Minerals
Antioxidants
Vitamins
Fiber
Natural water
Enzymes
phytonutrients
Unknown chemicals

Minerals

Your body contains around 4% minerals by weight.

Minerals have a lot functions in the body. Your body's growth and development depend on minerals. They act as partners with enzymes to work in your body to reduce inflammation. They provide structural support in bones and teeth, maintain water balance, are involved in muscle contraction and assist in enzyme function.

They combine with other molecules to form complex ions such as hemoglobin. They work to help **maintain alkaline-acid balance** throughout your entire body. And, they assist in the transmission of information from the brain to within all body systems.

You don't hear your mother saying, "take your minerals," normally you hear, "don't forget to take your vitamins, or eat your vegetables." But mineral are one step above vitamins in that many vitamins cannot do their job in your body without minerals.

There are two types of minerals. First, there are regular minerals such as calcium, sodium, phosphorous, magnesium, and potassium. These are the minerals you normally take daily.

Then there are trace minerals and these are like zinc, copper, arsenic, and iron. It's in the trace minerals that you can run the risk of mineral toxicity, since you don't need much of these trace minerals. Of course, there are more minerals in each category. Here is a list of the major minerals you find in fruits.

Sodium, potassium, chloride, calcium, phosphorus, magnesium, manganese
Here is a list of the trace minerals:

Iron, selenium, zinc, copper, iodide, fluoride, chromium, manganese, molybdenum, boron, nickel, silicon, arsenic, vanadium

Minerals are found both in meat and in fruits and vegetables. Our concentration here is on minerals found in fruits and how they can cure your body. Most all of these minerals are found in fruits, but there are some that are only found in meat and other foods.

There are other minerals that are called heavy metals. These tend to displace other beneficial minerals and cause toxic effects. These metals are:

Lead, cadmium, mercury, arsenic, iron

Vitamins

Vitamins are needed in small amounts in your body to help it perform normal functions, to provide for growth and to assist in body maintenance. There are two types of vitamins, fat soluble and water-soluble.

Most vitamins cannot be made in the body. Some can but in small amounts. For this reason, most vitamins that your body needs must come from the food you eat. Some fruits have vitamins, but they will not have all the vitamins your body needs.

Vitamins carry out various complex biochemical or physiological reactions in your body. When you lack the necessary vitamins your body needs, these chemical reactions do not occur often enough. The result is the creation of various illnesses. If the illnesses are not too far along, the illness can be reversed.

As with all illnesses, when it is not too far along, it can be reversed with the appropriate minerals, vitamins, or nutrients. In many cases, people wait too long before they address their illness. In many cases people don't know they are ill, or they just ignore that they don't feel good.

When it is reversible, then you need the foods that have the nutrients that will make you well and not the drugs that will keep or make you sick.

When you wait too long, when you have an illness, you get tissue damage in your organs, veins, arteries, or body that is not reversible using natural methods. Surgery or drugs can sometimes repair tissue damage, but you will not be the same as before when you were well.

This is one reason why having an alkaline body minimizes the tissue damage that you can get from an illness, since your will have less illness, when you have an alkaline body.

Fruits have a lot of different vitamins, but the level is rather low compared to the mineral content. The vitamins that fruits have are vitamin A and C in large quantities in some cases. They also have B-1, B-2, and niacin in low quantities.

Antioxidants

The body produces antioxidants to neutralize the free radicals that become excessive in your body. Free radicals have a damaging effect on the tissue they encounter as they float throughout your body. Left uncheck they cause numerous deadly diseases.

The way the body takes care of this threat is to create antioxidants. However, the body's antioxidants are not always enough to capture all the free radicals. This is because free radical can be created in numerous ways and can be found in food, air, water, and personal products.

Free radicals are also created with emotional states such as anger, fear, depression, and anxiety.

The result is that your body needs help to neutralize these free radicals, and this is where fruits come in. They are packed with antioxidants. Using them to neutralize free radicals has become a necessity.

There are many minerals and vitamins that are classified as antioxidants. These are vitamins A, C, E, and selenium. Other antioxidants are bioflavonoids, carotenoids, isoflavones, all minerals, allium vegetables like garlic and onions, bilberry, coenzyme Q10, cruciferous vegetables, ginkgo biloba, glutathione, lipoic acid, superoxide dismutase, and melatonin.

Antioxidants and Phytonutrients

Phytochemicals or phytonutrients are mostly found in the skin of fruits and are considered antioxidants. These nutrients give the fruit its color. Fruits also contain the fundamental antioxidants, vitamin A, C, E, beta carotene, zinc and selenium. Try to buy organic fruits so you can eat the skins without worry. In some fruits, there are more nutrients on the skin than in the fruit.

Other antioxidants that you may have heard of are

carotenoids, lutein, lycopene, sod, and glutathione, anthocyanins, and lipoic acid. The list is in the hundreds.

The discovery of antioxidants and their importance in preventing disease is one of the century's most important health discoveries. For this reason eating fruits and vegetables is probably the most important thing you can do, to prevent disease and improve your health.

Phytonutrients are special nutrients that are found in fruits and other plants. In plants, they protect them from disease, insects, excess heat, UV rays, poisons, pollutants, injury and drought.

Phytonutrients have been found to be beneficial to human life. They contain chemicals that are useful in treating and preventing diseases such as cancer, diabetes, cardiovascular disease, and hypertension.

The phytonutrients consists of many groups, but the most important groups are the phytosterols and phytohormones. These sterols are precursors to your human sterols.

Bioflavonoids

Bioflavonoids are also antioxidants that are chemicals, which come from water soluble colors found in fruits, vegetables, grains, leaves, and barks.

Because they are found in a variety of plant foods, they come in different chemical forms and concentrations.

Some of the bioflavonoids are more powerful in destroying free radicals then the standbys, vitamin C and E. Some well-known flavonoids are catechins, reserveratrol, and proanthocyanidines.

Enzymes

Enzymes are composed of different amino acids connected together. The body can create many enzymes, but not all, because it uses amino acids in its links and not all amino acids are created in your body. There are some amino acids that only come from the food you eat. So you need to eat certain foods to get the amino acids your body needs to create all the necessary enzymes.

Without enzyme activity in your body, you could not live. These chemical entities are required to help you breathe, give you energy, digest food, allow you to hear and see, and perform thousands of other body activities. There are over 75,000 of these enzymes in our body, and their chemical activity is constantly going on.

Enzymes are molecules that are catalysts. They start the chemical reaction of other molecules and compounds to produce the chemicals or functions that your body needs.

The body can only produce so many enzymes, and if you are sick, stressed, injured, depressed, or aged, then you will produce less. This will cause you to become even sicker.

You can also get enzymes from the raw food that you eat, which will supplement your body's enzymes. Enzymes are found in large quantities in raw fruits and vegetables. When food is processed and exposed to heat and encapsulated in a vacuum, the enzymes are destroyed.

All fruits have enzymes that help you digest them. This is why it is best to eat them raw so you can benefit from the natural enzymes. Eating fruits raw instead of cooked, in cans, in bottles, or in any other processed package saves your own body's enzymes. When your are sick, this help your immune system in that it does not have to use up its own enzymes, which are used up in fighting your disease. Enzymes are usually destroyed at about 115 deg F. That is why raw fruits are better for you than cooked fruits.

Your body has only a certain number of enzymes that it can produce in your life time. That is why after a certain age it is best to start taking digestive enzymes with each meal. But it is also wise to take digestive enzymes at any age.

Lack of digestive enzymes causes poor nutrition. Most elderly have poor nutrition and are very weak because they don't use digestive enzymes. In addition as you age, your stomach Hydrochloric acid, HCl, decreases and at some point in time you would need to supplement with digestive enzymes with HCl acid. You need good HCL in your stomach to transform some of the minerals and vitamins from the food you eat.

Laetrile

Laetrile is a vitamin called B17. Not much is said about it since it was once used in the US as a cancer drug, but it was banned because it contained small traces of arsenic.

Laetrile is found in apricots, apricot pits, cherries, and cherry pits. The laetrile in apricots and in cherries is not harmful. The pits should never be eaten because of the arsenic.

Free Radicals

When you eat fruits, your cells digest or metabolize the fruit nutrients and leave behind free radicals. Antioxidants neutralize these free radicals. Free radicals attack internal cell material, cell membrane, and tissue, creating inflammation and all kinds of diseases. Antioxidants are the main natural remedy for preventing arteriosclerosis, coronary heart disease, senility, aging, cancer, cataracts and many other inflammatory diseases.

Vary the fruits you eat because they vary in the type of antioxidants and nutrients that they have. Antioxidant levels are reduced in fruits when they are exposed to excess heat, sun, cooking, pressure, and packaging. Eat fruits of different colors because they contain different types of antioxidants.

Eat fruits when they turn ripe to get the right alkaline minerals into your body. When they are green, they produce acid in your body and when they are overripe, they contain too much sugar.

Fruit Chemicals Not Discovered Yet

Fruits have hundred of chemicals. Some are known and have been intensely studied. Others have yet to be discovered, and their purpose revealed. For this reason, it is best to eat a variety of fruits in the list given below, so that you can get the chemicals that can make you healthier, and that can cure any disease you might have.

11: Fruits That Cure When Drugs Don't

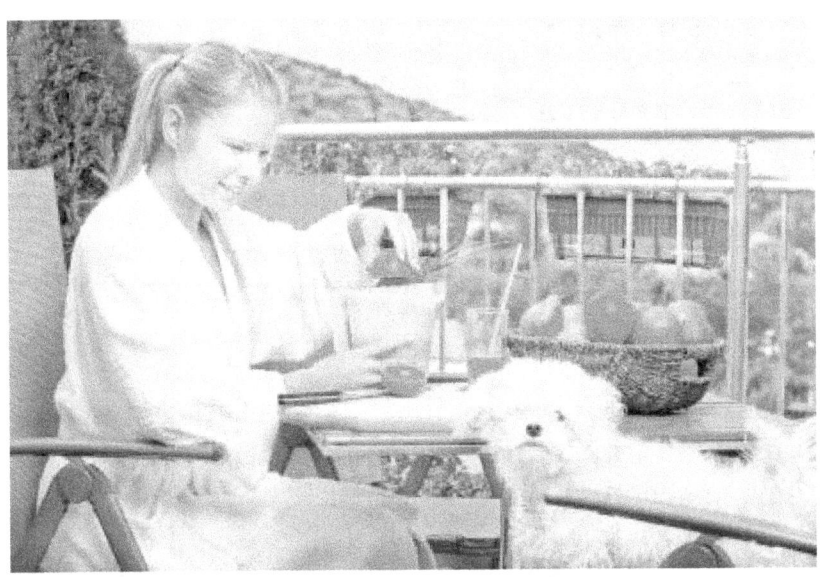

Natural Water

Your body consists of up to 70% or more of water. Fruits contain from 65% to 95% water. The water in your body is unique and in a condition that promotes many chemical reactions to take place for maintaining life. It is considered ionized water, since it has alkaline minerals in ionic form.

This ionic water allows many substances to dissolve. This water maintains your body temperature, and works as a lubricant for many body areas, including joints.

All fruits contain between 70-95% natural or distilled water. This is the best water your body can have. This composition is similar to the human body's water content. The muscles and brain contain 75% water, the blood 92%, bones 22%, and the overall body average is 60%.

Fruits That Cure

The fruits below are the fruits you should be eating. As you saw in the previous chapter, these fruits provide you a way to bind acid wastes in your body to give you perfect health.

In addition to their acid binding characteristics, fruits also play an important role in preventing, alleviating, or curing certain sickness or bodily symptom.

It is the combination of the nutrient within fruits that act together to perform curative bodily effects. In another previous chapter, you saw the different phytonutrients that fruits have. It's these phytonutrients, minerals, and vitamins that provide the anti-oxidants that reduce the amount of free radicals floating in your body that seek to damage tissue and organs.

There are no such things as being deficient in one mineral, vitamin, or nutrient. When there is a sickness, there may be one nutrient that is more lacking than others. But when you have a deficiency in one nutrient, you are surely deficient in many others. Nutrients always work together in your body.

When using fruits to help reach maximum health or to recover from an illness, it is best to use a combination of these fruits. Here is a list of the best fruits you should eat and use in combinations.

Apples – apples have been traditional being associated with relieving constipation and diarrhea and are still a good choice for these conditions. With their fiber and nutrients, they add bulk to your stools, making them easier to pass through your colon.

Eat one baked apple at night and one in the morning for constipation. For diarrhea, grate one apple, then let it sit for a couple of hours, until it darkens, then eat it. It is the pectin in apples that give it diarrhea curative effects.

The nutrients in apples are also effective in reducing the effects of stomach flu. For this, drink fresh apple juice or eat fresh apple sauce.

Apples have a high level of the fiber pectin, which is found mostly in its peel. Pectin has been found to be effective in controlling high cholesterol. It is also high in quercetin, an anti-oxidant, and vitamin C.

Dried apples with the peel are also good source pectin. Apples that have been canned or jarred have less pectin and have lost some of their anti-oxidant levels. But they still provide some nutrition.

Apricots – this fruit is a great source of beta-carotene, a nutrient that your body changes to vitamin A, and fiber. People who live long lives have a diet that consists of eating apricots when they are available.

Vitamin A has been associated with lower levels of cancer in people who eat and supplement with it regularly. It is also a good source of potassium and iron. For women who need more iron, apricots give them iron.

Dried apricots are high on the acid binding list, but only eat those that are organic and that don't use sulfur during dehydration.

In a stir fried chicken recipe, add organic dried apricots to add flavor, to soften them, and to offset the acid in the chicken.

Avocados – In a V.A. hospital in Coral Gables, people were fed one avocado a day and when blood samples were checked, these people showed a decrease in blood cholesterol of from 8% to 43%.

You can get relief from psoriasis, by eating 1/2 an avocado a day and then rubbing your skin with CamoCare cream. You get the oils from the avocado working internally and the cream working externally to help repair your skin.

Women in the Honduran Guatemalan border were

found to be using avocado oil on the face, hair, bodies to keep their skin from wrinkling and turning coarse from the hot sun and rough winds. Their use of this oil daily gave them a 10 to 20 year younger look.

Avocado and olive oil decrease the levels of bad cholesterol, LDL. Avocado has one of the best fats for your heath that you can find and not much is written about it – monounsaturated fat, omega-9.

Bananas – everyone loves bananas, and this is good because they are a good source of beta-carotene. It is known for its high level of potassium. It is also one of the only fruits that has the phytochemical fructoOligosaccharides, a fiber and vitamin B6, which feeds the good bacteria in your colon.

Studies have shown that potassium is good for high blood pressure. And, because of it high soluble fiber, it is also good for lowering cholesterol levels.

Banana peels have been found effective in removing all kinds of warts. The process is to take a ripe banana peel and cut out a section and place it over the wart and tape it down. Keep this on for two weeks or longer. Replace the peel when you shower or daily. As the days pass the wart will die by drying out and eventually will fall off.

When the elderly eat bananas daily, they appear to have better health and less sickness. Bananas are also good for offsetting the insulin shock experience by diabetics.

If you're a sports player or weight lifter, use bananas to gain weight that is reflected as muscle. If you need to gain weight, then eating two bananas a day will help you gain this weight.

If you have had too much liquor to drink, then do this. Take an organic banana peel and boil it, then drink the liquid. This will have a detoxifying effect on your body.

Berries – the berries cover here are all the different kinds of berries – currants, gooseberry, and strawberries. Nearly all berries are good for rejuvenating the blood and the heart. They have been found to reduce the risk of stroke by up to 40%.

All berries are a source of anti-cancer phytochemicals. They have vitamin C, fiber, and antioxidants, and many phytonutrients.

Berries have some degree of antiviral effects. For example, the poliovirus was found to be inactivated by a strawberry extract. Blueberries and cranberries reduce the activity of intestinal viruses and of the herpes simplex virus.
The currant berries contain a high level of Gamma Linolenic Acid, GLA, which gives relief to women during their premenstrual periods. Hypertension and arthritic inflammation are helped by using currants.

Gooseberries juice with some honey has been used for sore throats.

Strawberries and raspberries can be used in the prevention of tartar buildup on your teeth. Rub the berries onto your teeth and leave them on for as long as possible. This will prevent the buildup of tartar.

Strawberries are also a great facial cleaner. Here is a cream you can make:

Slightly heat 1 cup of almond oil and add 1/2 oz of beeswax and 1 tablespoon of lanolin. Add to this 1/2 cup of raw strawberry juice and mix well. Pour all of this into a jar and let set. When set, it is ready to use on your face.

Black Currant juice concentrate is high in vitamin C and flavonoids. These nutrients help to protect blood vessels and improve your eyesight.

Cantaloupe – this fruit has a high level of the antioxidant beta-carotene. With its high source of vitamin C, beta-carotene, potassium, doctors have discovered cantaloupe to be a protection from cancer of the esophagus.

Just half of cantaloupe can give you 800+ mg of potassium. This makes this fruit great for treating and maintaining normal blood pressure.

Melons are good as diuretics for bladder problems

and for constipation. Again, 1/2 a melon can activate a bowel movement within a couple of hours.

Watermelon seeds have been used as a diuretic for bladder infections. Fresh seeds are usually pounded to break them up and then boiled for 45 minutes to produce a liquid. After straining, this liquid is drunk 2 to 3 times a day.

The watermelon rind can be mashed up and used as a poultice, which is placed over the liver to relieve pain.

You can also create a cold watermelon drink by mixing watermelon with ice in a blender for a hot day.

By rubbing watermelon meat and rind on poison ivy, you can expect to get relief by the next day.

The best fruits to eat in the morning are watermelon, cantaloupes, and other melons. These give you the best alkaline ash residue to neutralize your body's acids. After your lemon drink, wait a while, take a shower and then cut up some melons. You can eat different melons and watermelons together, but do not mix them with other fruits. Eat melons on an empty stomach. You can eat them in between meals.

Cherries – cherries with their high level of antioxidants and a phytochemical called perillyl alcohol make it useful in protection against cancer. It has the ability to kill cancer cell without damage to good cells. Unfortunately, you cannot eat enough cherries for use against cancer.

The fiber and phytonutrients in cherries also make it a good remedy for constipation. By eating or drinking cherry juice between meals expect to become more regular.

If you ever have gout, then you want to eat cherries or drink cherry juice. Cherries are also good if you have arthritis, since cherries are high in antioxidants.

Citrus Fruits – Kumquat are also considered a citrus fruit. You can use them for high blood pressure and eat a couple after dinner. Wait about an hour before eating them.

Lemons - For bleeding gums, rub the rind part of a lemon along your bleeding gums each day. Uses as long as you have bleeding.

For a teeth whitening, use a combination of fresh lemon, lime, and grapefruit juice and brush your teeth and leave it on without rinsing your mouth. Do these three times a week.

For a toothache, use a cotton soak in lemon juice and put it on top or side of the aching tooth for a few minutes.

For a sore throat you can gargle with lemon juice a few times a day. This gargle can also be done with apples cider vinegar. Dilute the lemon or apple cider vinegar with water creating a 50:50 drink.

In the Acid Binding Fruit Chart, you will see that the fruit that gives you the best acid binding for your body is Lemon. It is high in potassium and calcium and is low in the minerals that produce acid – phosphorus, chlorine, and sulfur. Also notice it only takes 1 1/2 hours to digest, which helps you in the morning to detoxify your liver, blood and cells.

Here are different ways to use lemon in the morning, when you first wake up.

Squeeze one lemon juice into a glass of warm distilled water and drink up.

Squeeze one lemon juice into a glass, add one tablespoon of liquid chlorophyll, then add 6 – 8 oz of water and drink.

Put 6 oz. of water into a blender, squeeze one lemon juice without seeds. Add a pinch of cayenne pepper powder to increase the absorption and circulation of the nutrients. This will wake you up. Blend for about a minute and drink.

Whichever drink you use, after you finish rinse your mouth out with water to clean out the lemon acid from your mouth. This will protect your teeth enamel and prevent minerals from being brought in from your salvia to neutralize the lemon acids.

Lemons can be used for insomnia. Prepare a drink using lemon and orange juice, honey and hot water. Drink this just before going to bed.

Oranges and other citrus fruits - are good for breaking down fat. If you eat a few wedges of oranges after a fatty meal, this will help to break down the fat and allow you to process that fat easier through your body.

The vitamin C in oranges and in other citrus fruits is an anti-stress nutrient. It helps to detoxify your body by eliminating acid toxic wastes, repair cell damage, fight germs, and assists and strengthens your immune system.

Figs - Figs are a super food. They are high on the acid binding chart and one the foods with the highest fiber content.

Figs contain a substance called demulcents, which can sooth the irritated mucus membranes in your mouth, throat, and respiratory system.

For a sore throat, you can boil 3 or so figs in 4 cups of water for 4 to 6 minutes. Let the water cool then drink 1/4 cup every 3 to 4 hours.

For stomach ache and for constipation, eat figs between meals. Eat a few about an hour before bed time.

A research scientist, Jonathan L. Hartwell, discovered that figs affected different kinds of cancer. The active ingredient in figs that does this is benzaldehyde. For people that have cancer, eating figs is a good idea. Figs in and of themselves will not cure cancer, but they should be added to any treatment that is given to cancer patients.

Figs also have a phytochemical called ficin, which has been found useful in the treatment of chronic joint inflammation, rheumatoid arthritis and traumatic joint or muscle injuries.
A fig remedy for hemorrhoids is to boil fig leaves in water and apply this liquid to the anus. Since hemorrhoids are caused by constipation, you can also eat figs in the morning to help eliminate constipation.

Grapes – grapes are filled with phytochemicals. They contain resveratrol, ellagic acid, quercetin, and some phytosterols. Because of these phytochemicals, grapes are at the top of the list for fighting free radical. This also puts grapes at the top of the list for producing long life.

Doctors have found that drinking 10 ounces of purple grape juice a day will make blood platelets less sticky. This means blood clots, which can lead to heart attacks or strokes are less likely to occur. Grape juice is more effective than aspirin in reducing the formation of blood clots.

For the skin, use green Thompson seedless. Just cut

the grape slightly and rub the juice into the area where you want to reduce wrinkles. You can also blend these grapes and put this mash of grapes on your face and leave them on for 15 to 22 minutes.

Grapes contain traces of the mineral boron, which enhances brain activity. Use grapes every morning if possible to ensure good brain action.

Guavas – this fruit is high in lycopene, an antioxidant, and is a good source of Vitamin C. This fruit is great for lowering high blood pressure and cholesterol levels.

Ripe guavas can be used as a tonic for making weak hearts stronger. In addition, eating guavas helps to overcome lung and throat congestion.

Its juice has been used to control diabetes. Drink the juice right before a meal to control the sugar spikes that might come from that meal.

Mangoes - Mango and papaya are also high on the alkaline ash list so include them as snacks between meals. If you eat these after your morning lemon drink, you can eat melons as a snack before lunch.

For eye blood vessels that are weak due to diabetic retinopathy make a tea from mango leaves. Steep the leaves for an hour filter then combined with a couple of tablespoons of mango or pineapple. Now drink this combination.

Mango has been shown to be effective in giving constipation relief. Eat the mangos between meals. With the following fruit mixture, you can get rid of constipation and at the same time get maximum acid binding minerals into your body.

In a blinder put one banana, one mango, the juice of one lemon, and a bit of pineapple juice. You can use another acid binding fruit juice. Blend all ingredients and form a pudding.

Eat the sweet pudding and gain the benefits of all three fruits at one time. Do this every day and you will never have constipation.

For a facial mask to unclog pores and tighten your skin use a mashed up mango and put it on your face. The Papain in the mango will help to clean out your pores and surface skin. Try different times from 10 to 20 minutes to see what works best for you.

Papayas – this fruit contains a protein digestive enzyme called papain. Papain is available in tablets in many health food stores. It has been found that papain can neutralize snake poisons resulting from snake bites. By taking 5 tablets with 1 teaspoonful of Adolph's meat tenderizer dissolved in a cup of warm water within 30 minutes of a bite, a person has the chance of surviving a venous bite.

Cold sores inside and outside the mouth can also be cleared up by chewing on papain tablets.

Infected skin that has not responded to antibiotics can be cleared by putting fresh papayas on the wound for several hours.

When you have a chronic cough, eat papayas and mangos to get relief.

Peaches – Red peaches are a great source of beta-carotene coupled with vitamin C and fiber. Cooking peaches makes them loose a lot of their fiber.

If you want a facial mask made of peaches for skin rejuvenation, here's what to do. In a blender mix peach, papaya, banana and avocado, then place this mixture on your face for 30 minutes. Afterwards put some natural oil on your face like virgin coconut oil, or sunflower oil and expect better skin texture over time.

The leaves of a peach tree can be made into a tea to relieve morning sickness.
Use the peaches to give you fertility and long life.

Pears – are full of the insoluble fiber pectin. A single pear has 5 grams of fiber, and that's a lot, especially when your daily needs are around 25 to 35 grams.

Eat them in the morning and afternoon between meals to help you become more regular.

Pineapples – have the digestive enzyme bromelain.

Eating raw pineapples have been recommended for acute tendonitis. People with sports injuries also get relief when taking tablets of bromelain.

Bromelain is also useful for thinning the blood and improving blood circulation. Doctors use warfarin and coumadin to do just what bromelain does.

Pineapple has been used to get rid of warts and corns. Simply, by rubbing a slice of pineapple over a wart several times a day, the wart will fall off in a week or two.

Corns can be removed with pineapple. Tape a small piece of pineapple peel with the inside facing the corn. Leave it on overnight. The next day wash the area with hot water. Do the overnight application, until the corn comes off.

If you have ever experienced nausea from flying or riding on a boat, taking 8 oz. of pineapple or papaya juice will help to get rid of those feelings.

Pomegranates – the pomegranate seed has long been used to eliminate tapeworms. The way to use these seeds for tapeworms is to:

Dry the seed of 8 pomegranates in the sun or dehydrator

Crush the seed to a powder

Add to one glass of unsweetened pineapple juice

Drink this 3 times a day on an empty stomach.

Because pomegranates are loaded with vitamin C and antioxidants, they are great for sore throats, coughs, congestions and fevers.

Another remedy for sore throat is to boil the rind of the pomegranate and gargle with the liquid, after it cools.

Listed Fruits

The fruits listed above that you can eat are fantastic. Use them to remove acids from your body and to prevent or alleviate illness.

12: How Fruit Fiber Reduces Body Acids and Fight Diseases

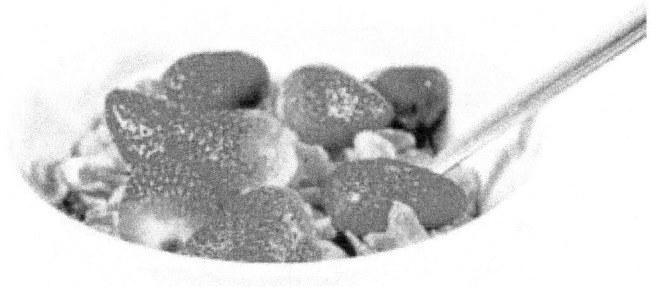

Fiber

All fruits contain fiber, some more than others. Fiber has many uses in the body. In the colon, it helps to prevent constipation, diverticulitis, hemorrhoids, and cancer and many other colon ills. Fiber pulls water into its structure as it goes through the intestines and colon, which softens the stool and makes it easier to pass through the colon.

If the food you have eaten does not have enough water, your stools will be hard and will have a difficult time moving through your colon. Then, if your stools sit in the colon too long, they will start to pull water out of your body, which can dehydrate you.

As fiber moves through the colon, it traps cholesterol, acids, toxins, carcinogens, estrogen, bile, **minerals**, and various un-digestible residues that come from the bile. Since, fiber traps cholesterol and many other un-needed nutrients, they will not be reabsorbed by the colon walls. This prevents unwanted nutrients from getting back into your body to create body acids.

Fiber also traps sugar into its fibers, allowing sugar to slowly be absorbed by the small intestine. This helps diabetics to process simple carbohydrates without experiencing an overdose of blood sugar. Slowing down the absorption of sugar, allows the diabetic to decrease the diabetic drug dose.

Fiber also provides food for the good bacteria, probiotics, which gives your colon health.

It is recommended that you have at least 25 to 35 mg of fiber every day, and up to 35 mg is better. Most people are eating around 8 to 12 mg every day. When you move from eating 10 mg to 25 mg, you may develop stomach gas, since your body is not used to processing a large increase in fiber. Just start increasing your fiber use slowly every day for a couple of weeks until you reach 25 – 35 mg.

It is not recommended to eat an excess of fiber, over 35 to 40 mg per day, since fiber also tends to tie up minerals, thus preventing them from being absorbed into your body.

There are two types of fiber – soluble and insoluble. Soluble fiber dissolves in water and forms a gooey and sticky mass. One type of soluble fiber is pectin. Pectin is found on the outside of some fruits like apples and pears and some is contained inside the fruit.

Soluble Fiber

Soluble Fiber becomes gummy and viscous, after it dissolves in water.

Soluble fiber has the ability to slow down digestion in the small intestine and prevent simple sugars from entering the bloodstream right away.

Because it absorbs water, soluble fiber softens and gives weight to fecal matter, and this makes fecal matter easier to pass through your colon.

Soluble fiber consists of pectin, gum, and mucilage. Pectin is found in carrots, apples, beets, cabbage, citrus fruits, and bananas. Gums and mucilage are found in oat bran, scsamc seeds, oats, oatmeal, legumes, guar gum, and gum Arabic.

Besides helping prevent constipation, soluble fiber provides the following benefits.

reduces the risk of heart disease
reduces the risk of gallstones

helps to remove toxic heavy metals and toxins from your colon
helps to prevent the toxic condition call appendicitis
regulates movement of sugar into the bloodstream
helps to prevent hemorrhoids and fissures
lowers cholesterol
lowers absorption of fats in the intestines and most importantly, helps prevent the overgrowth of bad bacteria in your colon.

Insoluble Fiber

Insoluble fiber does not dissolve in water and consists of cellulose, hemi cellulose, and lignin. This type of fiber is extremely beneficial to your health. Because your body's enzymes cannot break down this fiber, like it does food, it remains in tack as it travels through your intestines and colon.

Insoluble fiber helps the fecal matter travel faster through the small intestine and your colon.

It provides bulk to your fecal matter. It makes your stools larger, softer, and stimulates peristaltic movement as it touches your colon walls.

Insoluble fiber, like soluble fiber, slows down digestion. It also slows down absorption of protein, starch and fat and can inhibit the action of digestive enzymes.

Insoluble fiber is found in vegetables, wheat, and wheat bran. This type of fiber is considered an anti-carcinogen and a digestive aid. It is credited with preventing colon cancer and many other colon diseases.

Cellulose – Insoluble Fiber

Cellulose is a non-digestible carbohydrate which is found in the skins of fruits and vegetables – peas, green beans, carrots, broccoli, beets, brazil nuts, and lima beans.

Cellulose helps to remove cancer-causing toxins from your colon walls. It helps to prevent constipation, colitis, varicose veins, and hemorrhoids.

13: Breakfast Ideas That Stop Acids

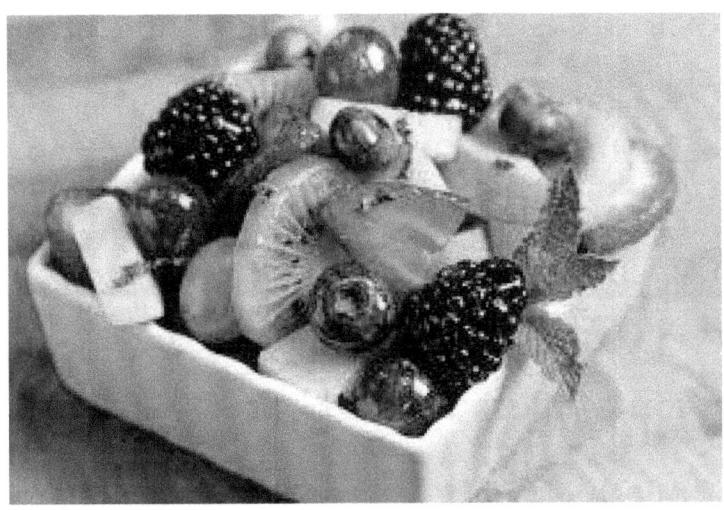

Breakfast

Here is a list of breakfast recipes that you can use, in the morning or any time you need a snack. These recipes can be used for cycle 1. Adjust the ingredients, for the number of people eating.

If you don't have some of the fruits in these recipes, use the ones you have.

Breakfast Pudding
   5 large dates, pitted
   1 apple, quartered and cored
   1 large frozen banana

Several sections of orange, to taste

Place all ingredients into a blender. Add a bit of apple juice, to get the blender started.

Peaches and Blueberries with a Melon Bowl
4 peaches, peeled and cubed
1 cup blueberries
2 small cantaloupes, halved and seeded

With a spoon or knife, cut up the cantaloupe into small pieces and place them in a bowl, with the other fruits.

Pumpkin Applesauce Pudding

1 cup applesauce
¾ cup pumpkin puree
¼ cup raisins
Ground cinnamon, to taste
Ground nutmeg, to taste
Ground allspice, to taste
Combine all the ingredients in a bowl.

Fruit Salad
Bananas
Kiwis
Mandarin oranges
Pineapple
Apples
Fresh lemon or lime juice

Cut up the fruits and place them in a bowl. You can use other fruits that are in season.

Smoothies

Apple Berry Smoothie
    1 cup apple juice
    2 apples, peeled, quartered, and cored
    ½ cup fresh or frozen blueberries
    ½ cup blackberries
    1 medium fresh or frozen banana
    2 dates, pitted
Blend all ingredients, in a blender for one minute.

Banana Peach Drink
    1 cup apple juice or orange juice
    1 large fresh or frozen banana
    2 ripe peaches, peeled, pitted, and cubed
    Fresh strawberries

Blend all ingredients, in a blender for one minute.

Coconut Smoothie
    1 cup regular or light coconut milk
    1 tablespoon maca powder
    1 tablespoon coconut oil
    1 tablespoon ground flax seeds
    1 teaspoon alcohol-free vanilla extract
    ¼ teaspoon almond extract
    ¼ teaspoon stevia powder
    8-10 ice cubes

Blend all ingredients, in a blender for one minute.

Fruit Shake
8 ounces orange or apple juice
1 medium banana
½ cup frozen diced peaches (purchased or frozen
fresh)

Use any other fruit or combination of fruits that you like.

Strawberry Banana Smoothie
3 cups fresh strawberries
2 medium frozen bananas
1 cup fresh young coconut water
2 tablespoons raw hulled hemp seeds or ground flax seeds.
Blend all ingredients, in a blender for one minute.

Snacks between Meals

Avocado Dressing
4-6 ripe medium avocados
¼ cup fresh lime juice
¼ cup fresh lemon juice
½ teaspoon powdered garlic
1/3 cup olive oil
Water, as needed for consistency
Salt and pepper, to taste

Mix all ingredients in a bowl until avocados is smooth

and not extra chunky.

Banana Avocado Snack
  2 medium bananas, sliced
  2 medium avocados, sliced
  Squeeze of fresh lemon or lime juice
  Salt to taste

Mix all ingredients in a bowl, until bananas and avocados are smooth and not extra chunky.

Guacamole
  8-10 ripe medium avocados
  2 tablespoons ground cumin
  1 tablespoon garlic, minced
  1 tablespoon ground coriander
  ¼ cup fresh lime juice
  1/8 cup fresh lemon juice
  2 large tomatoes, finely chopped

Mix all ingredients in a bowl, until avocados is smooth and not extra chunky. Cut this recipe down if you have less people to feed.

Tomato Basil Soup for Breakfast or Snack
  5 large tomatoes (about 2 pounds), quartered
  1 bunch fresh basil, chopped
  2 cups vegetable broth
  2 cloves garlic
  2 teaspoon olive oil
  2 tablespoons balsamic vinegar
  Salt and pepper, to taste

Avocado chunks or sautéed eggplant, for garnish

You can eat this hot or cold. If you want to eat it hot, place all these ingredients into a pot and heat for 10 minutes.

Salads
California Morning Salad
1 somewhat firm avocado, diced
1 cucumber, diced
1 jalapeño chile pepper, sliced into thin rings
1 (3.8-ounce) can sliced olives
Juice from 1 lemon
Juice from 1 lime
¼ cup olive oil

Mix all ingredients into a bowl and toss.

Grapefruit with Avocado Salad
1 grapefruit, cut into segments and ¼ cup juice reserved
1 avocado, sliced or diced
¼ cup olive oil
¼- ½ teaspoon kosher salt
1 teaspoon Dijon mustard
Black pepper and black salt, to taste

Mix in a bowl and eat for breakfast or as a snack.

Banana Breakfast Pudding
1 medium ripe banana

6 dates, soaked in water for up to 30 minutes
2 to 3 peaches, pitted, or meat and water from 1
young coconut
2 teaspoon alcohol-free vanilla extract
1 teaspoon ground cinnamon
Agave nectar, to taste

Blend all Ingredients

14: About The Author And Other Resources

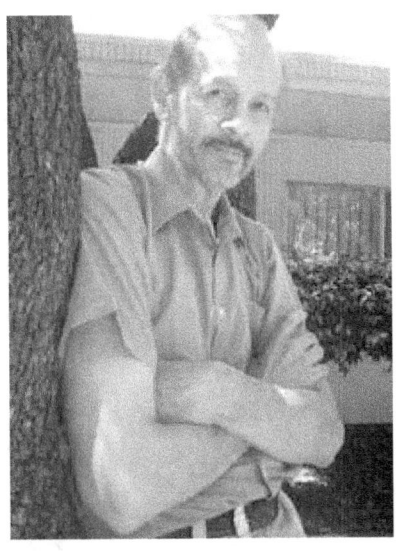

Rudy Silva is a natural consultant nutritionist educated in the United States in Nutrition and Physics. He is a graduate from the San Jose State University in California. He is author of 30 other e-books on natural remedies. He has authored a newsletter in natural remedies for over 4 years. He has many websites promoting special recommended products and information.

Resource page

Here are some of the other kindle e-books about natural remedies that have been written by this author. You can see the entire list at:

http://tinyurl.com/b2f7wd3

Acne Remedies
Best natural acne treatments: Acne facial

Constipation Remedies
Best Constipated Women Natural Cures
Natural Constipation Remedies:

Essential Fatty Acids
Taking The Mystery Out Of Essential Fatty acids

Nutrition Remedies
Fast Healing Juice Nutrition Therapy: Nutrition Tips 3
Fantastic Alkaline Fruit Benefits Revealed
Calcium (Discover How To Use Calcium To Avoid Devastating Diseases)
Magnesium Nutrition Revealed
Potassium Health Secrets Revealed
Phosphorus, The Best Brain Food
A Sodium Diet (What You Must Know About Sodium)
Calcium and Magnesium Magic Body Benefits Revealed

Stomach Remedies
Acid Reflux: Fast and Easy Cures For Acid Reflux
How To Do Natural Colon Cleansing

Misc. Remedies
Natural Hair Loss Treatment: Women And Men
Effective Natural Hemorrhoids Treatment
Iron Deficiency Anemia
Best Impotence Health Diet

Men's Health
Best Impotence Health Diet

Weight loss
Ten (10) Day Quick Success Weight Loss Program: A new approach to losing weight by changing your eating habits for life.

To see all of the kindle books written by this author, go to this the Authors Profile Page or this URL:

http://tinyurl.com/b2f7wd3

If you need support or want to promote any of his e-books, please contact him at rss41@yahoo.com and expect a reply within 24 hours. He looks forward to hearing from you and is happy to help you understand his material on natural and nutritional health.

Give A Review

And, don't forget to give a review for this e-book at Amazon so that others can gain the benefits of what is in this e-book. It can be a one or two sentence review.

To you, for losing weight, creating better health and more happiness in your life,

Rudy S Silva

www.ingramcontent.com/pod-product-compliance
Lightning Source LLC
Chambersburg PA
CBHW060413290526
45791CB00002B/730